STAYING PHYSICALLY FIT AT 50 AND BEYOND

"Transform Your Body, Transform Your Life: Fitness After 50."

ANTHONY ODITA

First Edition: October 2020

ISBN:

Published

Published by Anthony Odita

Anthony Odita Publications

+234-8143375192

Sought After Believers Ministry International

Sabministry@gmail.com

Email: oditaanthony@yahoo.com

Dedication

To everyone striving to stay active, strong, and vibrant at every age.

This book is dedicated to those who view aging not as a limitation but as an opportunity to grow, challenge, and reinvent themselves. May this journey inspire you to embrace wellness, celebrate movement, and find joy in each new day.

Here's to a lifetime of vitality, at 50 and beyond.

Table Of Contents

Introduction

As we reach our 50s and beyond, staying physically fit becomes more important than ever. It's a time to embrace new challenges, redefine our health, and unlock a vibrant lifestyle. This book is designed to guide you through the essential aspects of fitness tailored specifically for this stage of life.

In these pages, you'll discover practical strategies for assessing your current fitness level, creating a balanced workout plan, and making informed nutritional choices. You'll also find motivation and support to overcome common barriers, along with effective exercise routines suited to various fitness levels.

Whether you're just beginning your fitness journey or looking to refine your existing regimen, "Staying Physically Fit At 50 And Beyond" will empower you to take charge of your health and enjoy a fulfilling, active life. Let's embark on this journey together and embrace the possibilities that come with age!

Chapter 1:
Assessing Your Fitness Level

Assessing your current fitness level is a crucial first step in your journey to staying physically fit at 50 and beyond. Understanding where you stand allows you to set realistic goals, track your progress, and tailor your exercise plan to meet your unique needs. In this chapter, we will explore various methods to evaluate your fitness, identify your strengths and weaknesses, and establish a baseline for future improvement.

1.1 Fitness Assessments

To accurately assess your fitness level, consider conducting the following evaluations:

Cardiovascular Endurance: A simple way to gauge your endurance is through a walking or running test. Measure how long it takes to cover a specific distance, such as a mile, or track your heart rate recovery after exercise.

Muscular Strength: You can test your strength through exercises like push-ups, squats, or a grip strength test using a dynamometer. Record how many repetitions you can perform or measure the maximum weight you can lift for a specific exercise.

Flexibility: The sit-and-reach test is a common measure of flexibility. Sit on the floor with your legs extended, and reach toward your toes to see how far you can go. This will help assess flexibility in your lower back and hamstrings.

Body Composition: Understanding your body composition—specifically your body fat percentage versus lean muscle mass—can provide insights into your overall health. You can use calipers, bioelectrical impedance scales, or professional assessments for accurate readings.

1.2 Identifying Strengths and Weaknesses

After conducting your assessments, take time to analyze the results. Consider the following:

Strengths: What exercises or activities do you excel at? Recognizing your strengths can help you build confidence and incorporate them into your routine.

Weaknesses: Identify areas where you may struggle. This could include low endurance, limited strength, or lack of flexibility. Acknowledging these weaknesses is essential for creating a balanced fitness plan that addresses them.

1.3 Creating a Baseline for Progress

Once you've assessed your fitness level, it's time to establish a baseline. Document your results, noting specific numbers and observations. This baseline will serve as a reference point to track your progress over time. Regular reassessment—every few months or as you progress—will help you see improvements, adjust your fitness plan, and keep you motivated.

By understanding your current fitness level, you are better equipped to set achievable goals, design a personalized fitness plan, and embark on a successful journey toward staying physically fit at 50 and beyond.

Remember, every step you take toward fitness is a step toward a healthier, more vibrant life!

Chapter 2:
Creating a Balanced Fitness Plan

A balanced fitness plan is essential for maintaining health and vitality as you age. It should address all components of fitness, including cardiovascular endurance, muscular strength, flexibility, and balance. In this chapter, we will explore how to create a personalized fitness plan that fits your lifestyle, goals, and abilities.

2.1 Types of Exercise

To achieve a well-rounded fitness routine, incorporate the following types of exercise:

Cardiovascular Exercise: Aim for at least 150 minutes of moderate-intensity or 75 minutes of vigorous-intensity aerobic activity each week. This can include walking, jogging, swimming, cycling, or dancing. Choose activities you enjoy to make it easier to stick with your routine.

Strength Training: Include strength training exercises at least two days a week. Focus on major muscle groups using bodyweight exercises, resistance bands, free weights, or weight machines. This will help maintain muscle mass, support bone health, and boost metabolism.

Flexibility and Stretching: Incorporate flexibility exercises into your routine to improve range of motion and reduce the risk of injury. Aim to stretch major muscle groups at least two to three times a week, holding each stretch for 15-30 seconds.

Balance Exercises: As we age, maintaining balance is crucial for preventing falls. Include balance training exercises, such as standing on one leg or practicing tai chi, at least two to three times a week.

2.2 Balancing Cardio and Strength Training

When creating your fitness plan, it's essential to strike a balance between cardiovascular and strength training. A well-rounded routine might look like this:

Weekly Schedule Example:

Monday: 30 minutes of brisk walking + 20 minutes of strength training (upper body)

Tuesday: 30 minutes of cycling or swimming

Wednesday: Rest or light activity (yoga, stretching)

Thursday: 30 minutes of brisk walking + 20 minutes of strength training (lower body)

Friday: 30 minutes of dancing or aerobics

Saturday: Balance and flexibility exercises (yoga or tai chi)

Sunday: Rest or light activity

Feel free to adjust the schedule to fit your preferences and commitments. The key is consistency and gradually increasing the intensity and duration of your workouts as your fitness level improves.

2.3 Crafting a Weekly Workout Schedule

To make your fitness plan manageable and enjoyable, create a weekly workout schedule that includes:

Specific Days and Times: Set aside dedicated time for each workout, treating it like an important appointment. This helps establish a routine.

Variety: Include different types of exercises to keep things interesting. Mixing up your workouts will help prevent boredom and reduce the risk of injury.

Rest Days: Ensure you incorporate rest days to allow your body to recover. Recovery is crucial for muscle repair and overall progress.

Listen to Your Body: Pay attention to how your body responds to your workouts. If you feel fatigued or experience pain, consider modifying your routine or allowing for additional rest.

By creating a balanced fitness plan tailored to your unique needs and goals, you'll set yourself up for success as you strive to stay physically fit at 50 and beyond. Remember, the journey to fitness is a personal one—embrace it, enjoy it, and celebrate your progress along the way!

Chapter 3:
Nutrition Essentials for Vitality

Nutrition plays a crucial role in maintaining health and vitality as we age. Proper dietary choices can enhance energy levels, support physical performance, and help prevent chronic diseases. In this chapter, we'll explore the essential components of a nutritious diet tailored for individuals aged 50 and beyond.

3.1 Understanding Nutritional Needs After 50

As we age, our bodies undergo various changes that affect nutritional needs. Here are key considerations:

Caloric Needs: Metabolism tends to slow down with age, leading to decreased caloric requirements. It's essential to focus on nutrient-dense foods rather than empty calories to ensure adequate nutrition without excess weight gain.

Protein: Adequate protein intake is vital for preserving muscle mass and strength. Aim for about 0.8 to 1.0 grams of protein per kilogram of body weight. Include lean meats, fish, eggs, dairy, legumes, and plant-based protein sources.

Calcium and Vitamin D: These nutrients are critical for bone health, especially for postmenopausal women. Aim for 1,200 mg of calcium and 800-1,000 IU of vitamin D daily. Sources include dairy products, fortified foods, leafy greens, and sun exposure for vitamin D.

Fibre: High fibre intake is essential for digestive health and can help manage weight. Aim for at least 25 grams of fiber per day from whole grains, fruits, vegetables, legumes, and nuts.

Hydration: As we age, our sense of thirst may diminish, making hydration a priority. Aim to drink at least 8 cups (64 ounces) of water daily, adjusting for physical activity and climate.

3.2 Meal Planning and Preparation

Creating nutritious meals requires planning and preparation. Here are some strategies:

Balanced Plates: Strive for a balanced plate that includes a variety of food groups:

Half the Plate: Fill half your plate with colourful fruits and vegetables. They provide essential vitamins, minerals, and antioxidants.

One-Quarter of the Plate: Include lean proteins such as chicken, fish, tofu, or beans.

One-Quarter of the Plate: Add whole grains like brown rice, quinoa, or whole-wheat pasta.

Meal Prep: Dedicate time each week to plan and prepare meals. Batch cooking, pre-chopping vegetables, and portioning snacks can save time and promote healthier eating choices.

Mindful Eating: Pay attention to portion sizes and eat slowly. This practice can help prevent overeating and increase enjoyment of your meals.

3.3 Supplements: What You Need to Know

While a balanced diet should provide most nutrients, supplements may be beneficial for some individuals. Consider the following:

Consult a Healthcare Provider: Before starting any supplements, consult with your healthcare provider to assess your individual needs and avoid potential interactions with medications.

Common Supplements: Some nutrients that may require supplementation include:

Vitamin D: Especially for those with limited sun exposure.

Calcium: If dietary intake is insufficient.

Omega-3 Fatty Acids: For heart and brain health, particularly if you don't consume fish regularly.

Avoid Over-Reliance on Supplements: Remember that supplements are meant to complement a healthy diet, not replace it. Focus on whole foods first.

By understanding and implementing these nutrition essentials, you can enhance your vitality and support your overall health as you age. Making informed dietary choices empowers you to lead an active and fulfilling life at 50 and beyond. Remember, nourishing your body is one of the most significant investments you can make in your health and well-being!

Chapter 4:
Staying Motivated

Maintaining motivation is a crucial aspect of any fitness journey, especially as we age. The enthusiasm you feel at the beginning can sometimes wane, but with the right strategies and mindset, you can keep your motivation high and continue making progress. In this chapter, we'll explore effective ways to stay motivated in your fitness routine and overcome common obstacles.

4.1 Finding Your "Why"

Understanding your personal reasons for staying fit is fundamental to sustaining motivation. Take time to reflect on what drives you. Some common motivations might include:

Improving Health: Reducing the risk of chronic diseases, improving cardiovascular health, or managing weight.

Enhancing Quality of Life: Increasing energy levels, enhancing mobility, or improving mental clarity and mood.

Setting an Example: Being a role model for family and friends or inspiring others to lead healthier lifestyles.

Write down your motivations and keep them visible. Revisiting these reasons can reignite your passion when you feel your motivation slipping.

4.2 Setting Realistic and Achievable Goals

Setting specific, measurable, achievable, relevant, and time-bound (SMART) goals can provide direction and purpose. Here's how to do it:

Specific: Clearly define what you want to achieve. Instead of saying, "I want to be fit," specify, "I want to walk 30 minutes five days a week."

Measurable: Make sure your goals can be tracked. Use fitness apps, journals, or wearable devices to log your workouts and progress.

Achievable: Set goals that are challenging yet attainable. Consider your current fitness level and any physical limitations.

Relevant: Ensure your goals align with your motivations and lifestyle. They should be meaningful to you personally.

Time-Bound: Establish a timeframe for your goals. Setting deadlines can create a sense of urgency and accountability.

4.3 Dealing with Setbacks

Setbacks are a normal part of any journey, and learning to navigate them is key to staying motivated. Here are some strategies:

Expect Challenges: Understand that obstacles will arise, whether it's an injury, illness, or life changes. Acknowledging this helps you prepare mentally.

Stay Flexible: Be willing to adapt your fitness routine when necessary. If you can't run, consider walking or swimming instead. The goal is to keep moving, even if it's not your preferred activity.

Practice Self-Compassion: Don't be too hard on yourself when setbacks occur. Remind yourself that it's okay to have off days and that progress is not always linear.

4.4 Building a Support Network

Surrounding yourself with supportive individuals can significantly enhance motivation:

Workout Partners: Find a friend, family member, or group to exercise with. Shared goals and accountability can make workouts more enjoyable.

Community Groups: Join local fitness classes, clubs, or online forums. Engaging with others who share similar goals can provide encouragement and camaraderie.

Professional Guidance: Consider working with a personal trainer or joining a fitness program designed for your age group. Professionals can offer expertise, motivation, and tailored workouts.

4.5 Celebrating Milestones

Recognizing and celebrating your achievements, no matter how small, is essential for maintaining motivation:

Track Progress: Regularly assess your fitness improvements, whether it's increased endurance, strength gains, or weight loss.

Reward Yourself: Treat yourself to non-food rewards for reaching milestones, such as new workout gear, a spa day, or a special outing.

Reflect on Your Journey: Take time to look back at how far you've come. Reflecting on your journey can rekindle your motivation and inspire continued efforts.

Staying motivated is an ongoing process, but by identifying your reasons, setting achievable goals, navigating setbacks, building a support network, and celebrating your successes, you can maintain your **enthusiasm for fitness.** Embrace the journey of staying physically fit at 50 and beyond, and remember that every step you take is a step toward a healthier, more vibrant life!

Chapter 5:

Effective Exercise Routines

Creating effective exercise routines is essential for achieving your fitness goals, especially as you navigate the unique challenges and changes that come with age. A well-rounded routine includes cardiovascular, strength, flexibility, and balance exercises tailored to your fitness level. In this chapter, we will explore various types of effective exercise routines to keep you engaged and motivated.

5.1 Beginner-Friendly Workouts

If you're new to exercising or returning after a long break, start with beginner-friendly routines that focus on building a solid foundation. Here are some options:

Walking: Aim for 20-30 minutes of brisk walking at least five times a week. Walking is low-impact and can be done anywhere.

Bodyweight Exercises: Start with simple bodyweight exercises that can be performed at home. Focus on:

Squats: 2 sets of 8-10 repetitions

Modified Push-Ups: 2 sets of 5-10 repetitions (use a wall or a bench for support)

Seated Leg Lifts: 2 sets of 10-12 repetitions (while seated in a chair)

Flexibility Routine: Incorporate gentle stretching exercises to improve flexibility. Hold each stretch for 15-30 seconds and target major muscle groups, such as hamstrings, quadriceps, shoulders, and back.

5.2 Intermediate Challenges

Once you feel comfortable with the basics, consider incorporating more challenging exercises into your routine:

Interval Training: Alternate between moderate and higher intensity in your cardio workouts. For example, walk briskly for two minutes, then increase your pace for one minute, and repeat for 20-30 minutes.

Strength Training with Weights: Use dumbbells or resistance bands to enhance strength. Aim for 2-3 sessions per week, including:

Dumbbell Shoulder Press: 3 sets of 10-12 repetitions

Lunges: 3 sets of 8-10 repetitions per leg

Bent-Over Rows: 3 sets of 10-12 repetitions

Balance Exercises: Include exercises like heel-to-toe walking, single-leg stands, or yoga poses (e.g., tree pose) to improve stability and coordination.

5.3 Advanced Fitness Techniques

For those who are already active and looking for new challenges, consider the following advanced techniques:

High-Intensity Interval Training (HIIT): Incorporate short bursts of intense activity followed by brief recovery periods. An example routine could include:

30 seconds of jumping jacks, followed by 30 seconds of rest, repeated for 20 minutes.

Circuit Training: Combine strength and cardio exercises in a circuit format. Create a routine with 5-6 different exercises (e.g., squats, push-ups, jumping jacks, planks) and perform each for 30 seconds to 1 minute with minimal rest in between.

Group Classes: Join fitness classes such as spinning, kickboxing, or yoga. These classes provide structure, expert guidance, and a supportive community.

5.4 Sample Weekly Workout Routine

To illustrate how to incorporate various elements of fitness, here's a sample weekly workout routine:

Monday: 30 minutes of brisk walking + 20 minutes of strength training (upper body)

Tuesday: 30 minutes of interval training (e.g., alternating walking and jogging)

Wednesday: Rest or light activity (gentle yoga or stretching)

Thursday: 30 minutes of cycling + 20 minutes of strength training (lower body)

Friday: 30 minutes of group fitness class (e.g., aerobics or Zumba)

Saturday: Balance and flexibility exercises (yoga or tai chi)

Sunday: Rest or leisurely outdoor activity (hiking or gardening)

5.5 Listening to Your Body

As you engage in exercise routines, it's essential to listen to your body. Pay attention to how you feel during and after workouts:

Modify as Needed: If you experience pain or discomfort, consider modifying exercises or choosing lower-impact alternatives.

Rest When Necessary: Allow for adequate recovery time between workouts, especially after intense sessions. Rest is crucial for muscle repair and overall health.

Celebrate Progress: Track your achievements, no matter how small. Celebrate milestones, such as increasing weights or completing a challenging workout.

Creating effective exercise routines that align with your fitness level and goals is key to staying physically fit at 50 and beyond. Remember that consistency is more important than intensity; focus on making movement a regular part of your life, and enjoy the journey toward better health and vitality!

Chapter 6:
Mindfulness and Recovery

Incorporating mindfulness and recovery practices into your fitness regimen is essential for enhancing overall well-being, promoting mental clarity, and facilitating physical recovery. As we age, the importance of taking care of our minds and bodies becomes even more apparent. In this chapter, we'll explore various mindfulness techniques and recovery strategies to help you stay physically fit and balanced.

6.1 The Importance of Mindfulness

Mindfulness involves being present in the moment and fully engaged with your thoughts, feelings, and sensations. This practice can enhance your fitness journey in several ways:

Reducing Stress: Mindfulness helps lower stress levels, which can negatively impact physical health. Techniques such as deep breathing, meditation, and guided imagery can promote relaxation.

Improving Focus: Mindfulness enhances your ability to concentrate during workouts. Being present allows you to perform exercises with better form and technique, reducing the risk of injury.

Encouraging Healthy Choices: Practicing mindfulness can lead to greater awareness of your body's needs, helping you make healthier food and exercise choices.

6.2 Mindfulness Techniques

Here are some mindfulness techniques you can incorporate into your daily routine:

Breathing Exercises: Spend a few minutes focusing on your breath. Inhale deeply through your nose, allowing your abdomen to expand, then exhale slowly through your mouth. Repeat this process for several minutes to cultivate calmness.

Meditation: Set aside time each day for meditation. Find a quiet space, sit comfortably, and focus on your breath or a specific mantra. Start with just five minutes and gradually increase the duration.

Body Scan: This technique involves mentally scanning your body for tension. Start at your toes and move up to your head, paying attention to how each part feels. Release any tension you notice as you breathe deeply.

Mindful Walking: While walking, focus on each step you take. Pay attention to the sensations in your feet, the rhythm of your breath, and the sights and sounds around you. This practice combines physical activity with mindfulness.

6.3 Recovery Techniques

Recovery is just as important as exercise for maintaining fitness, especially as we age. Proper recovery techniques help reduce soreness, prevent injuries, and promote overall well-being:

Active Recovery: Engage in low-intensity activities on rest days, such as walking, gentle yoga, or swimming. These activities promote blood flow and aid recovery without putting additional strain on your body.

Stretching: Incorporate stretching into your routine to improve flexibility and reduce muscle tightness. Focus on major muscle groups and hold each stretch for at least 15-30 seconds.

Hydration: Staying hydrated is vital for recovery. Drink plenty of water before, during, and after workouts to replenish fluids lost through sweat.

Nutrition: Proper nutrition supports recovery. Focus on a balanced diet that includes lean proteins, healthy fats, whole grains, and a variety of fruits and vegetables. Post-workout meals should include protein and carbohydrates to aid muscle repair.

Sleep: Prioritize quality sleep, as it is crucial for recovery and overall health. Aim for 7-9 hours of sleep per night and establish a consistent sleep routine.

6.4 Listening to Your Body

Mindfulness and recovery practices encourage you to tune into your body's signals. Here are some ways to ensure you're listening effectively:

Recognize Fatigue: Pay attention to signs of fatigue or overtraining. If you feel excessively tired or sore, consider taking a rest day or adjusting your workout intensity.

Adjust Goals as Needed: Your fitness journey is a dynamic process. Be open to adjusting your goals based on how you feel physically and mentally.

Celebrate Small Wins: Acknowledge and celebrate your progress, no matter how small. Mindfulness can help you appreciate each step in your journey, enhancing motivation and satisfaction.

Chapter 7:
Active Living Beyond the Gym

Staying physically fit doesn't have to be confined to the gym. In fact, incorporating physical activity into your daily life can be just as beneficial, if not more so, than structured workouts. In this chapter, we'll explore various ways to stay active outside of the gym, emphasizing the importance of an active lifestyle for overall health and well-being.

7.1 Embracing Everyday Activities

Engaging in everyday activities can significantly contribute to your fitness without the need for formal exercise sessions. Consider the following:

Walking or Biking: Choose walking or biking instead of driving for short trips. Incorporate walking meetings or bike rides into your routine to make errands more active.

Household Chores: Turn chores into a workout! Vacuuming, gardening, washing the car, and yard work can elevate your heart rate and strengthen muscles.

Active Commuting: If possible, consider walking or biking to work. If you use public transportation, get off one stop early and walk the rest of the way.

Taking the Stairs: Opt for stairs instead of elevators or escalators. Climbing stairs is an excellent way to build strength and improve cardiovascular fitness.

7.2 Exploring Outdoor Activities

Nature offers a variety of opportunities for staying active. Here are some outdoor activities to consider:

Hiking: Explore local trails and parks. Hiking not only provides a great workout but also allows you to connect with nature and enjoy the outdoors.

Walking Clubs: Join a walking group in your community. This social activity can make walking more enjoyable and provide motivation.

Playing Sports: Engage in recreational sports such as tennis, golf, or swimming. These activities are fun and help improve coordination and cardiovascular health.

Gardening: Gardening is an excellent form of physical activity that involves bending, lifting, and digging. It also has mental health benefits, promoting relaxation and mindfulness.

7.3 Incorporating Movement into Leisure Time

Finding ways to stay active during leisure time can keep you engaged and promote a healthier lifestyle:

Active Hobbies: Choose hobbies that involve physical activity, such as dancing, cycling, or martial arts. These activities can be both enjoyable and beneficial for fitness.

Family Activities: Plan active outings with family and friends, such as bowling, mini-golf, or hiking. Involving loved ones can make physical activity a social event.

Volunteer Opportunities: Look for volunteer opportunities that require physical activity, such as helping at a local animal shelter or participating in community clean-up events.

7.4 Staying Mindful of Movement

Incorporating movement into your daily life requires awareness and intention. Here are some tips to help you stay mindful of your activity levels:

Set Daily Movement Goals: Aim for a certain number of steps each day or designate time for physical activity. Tracking your movement can help keep you accountable.

Use Technology: Consider using a fitness tracker or smartphone app to monitor your daily activity levels. These tools can provide motivation and insights into your habits.

Schedule Movement Breaks: If you have a sedentary job, set a timer to remind you to stand up, stretch, or take a short walk every hour. This can help prevent stiffness and fatigue.

7.5 Balancing Rest and Activity

While staying active is crucial, it's equally important to balance activity with rest:

Listen to Your Body: Pay attention to how your body feels. If you're tired or experiencing discomfort, allow yourself time to rest and recover.

Restorative Activities: Incorporate restorative practices such as yoga, stretching, or meditation into your routine to promote relaxation and recovery.

Prioritize Sleep: Quality sleep is essential for overall health. Aim for 7-9 hours of sleep each night to support your physical and mental well-being.

Active living beyond the gym is an empowering approach to maintaining fitness and overall health. By embracing everyday activities, exploring outdoor adventures, and incorporating movement into your leisure time, you can create a vibrant and active lifestyle that enhances your well-being as you age. Remember, fitness is not just about structured workouts; it's about cultivating a life full of movement and joy!

Conclusion

Staying physically fit at 50 and beyond is not only achievable but incredibly rewarding. This journey involves more than simply exercising; it's about embracing a lifestyle that nourishes your body, mind, and spirit. By assessing your fitness level, setting realistic goals, and following a balanced fitness plan, you're taking meaningful steps toward a healthier, more vibrant life.

From nutrition and exercise routines to mindfulness and active living, each chapter of this book provides tools and strategies designed to empower you at every stage of your fitness journey. Recovery and self-care practices are just as crucial as workouts, helping you sustain energy, reduce injury risks, and stay motivated for the long haul.

As you've discovered, fitness goes beyond the walls of the gym. Active living, engaging with your environment, and finding joy in movement can deeply enrich your daily life. Embracing this holistic approach to fitness allows you to cultivate strength, flexibility, and resilience, not just in your body, but in your outlook as well.

Remember that every step forward, no matter how small, contributes to your overall wellness. Celebrate your progress, adjust as needed, and prioritize what brings you joy and vitality. Fitness is a lifelong commitment, and the benefits extend far beyond physical health—they encompass mental clarity, emotional resilience, and a greater zest for life. Here's to thriving at 50 and beyond—because this is just the beginning!

Resources

Here are some recommended resources to support you on your journey to staying physically fit and healthy beyond 50. These resources include books, websites, and apps focused on fitness, nutrition, mindfulness, and overall wellness.

Books

"Younger Next Year: Live Strong, Fit, and Sexy - Until You're 80 and Beyond" by Chris Crowley and Henry S. Lodge

An inspiring guide with practical tips for staying active, healthy, and vibrant in later years.

"The Joy of Movement" by Kelly McGonigal, PhD

This book explores the psychological benefits of exercise and how movement can bring joy and resilience to your life.

"Strength Training Past 50" by Wayne L. Westcott and Thomas R. Baechle

A detailed guide on strength training specifically for older adults, offering exercises and advice tailored to aging bodies.

"The Complete Guide to Food and Nutrition for Older Adults" by Roberta Larson Duyff

A comprehensive guide to understanding and managing your nutrition as you age, with tips for optimizing diet and health.

Websites

National Institute on Aging (NIA)

www.nia.nih.gov

This government site offers a wide range of health, wellness, and exercise resources for older adults.

ChooseMyPlate.gov

www.choosemyplate.gov

A useful resource for dietary guidelines, meal planning, and portion control tips, specifically tailored for various age groups.

American Council on Exercise (ACE)

www.acefitness.org

The ACE website provides information on exercise routines, fitness assessments, and tips for different age groups.

Mindful.org

www.mindful.org

This site offers articles, guided meditations, and resources on incorporating mindfulness practices into daily life.

Apps

MyFitnessPal

A versatile app for tracking nutrition and exercise, offering an extensive food database and personalized goals.

Headspace

Known for its guided meditations, Headspace can help with incorporating mindfulness and relaxation into your routine.

MapMyWalk / MapMyRun

These apps by Under Armour are perfect for tracking walking, running, and other outdoor activities, providing data on distance, pace, and routes.

SilverSneakers GO

An app designed for seniors, offering workouts, fitness schedules, and videos tailored to different fitness levels.

FitOn

A free app with workout videos in various categories, including strength, cardio, and stretching, led by trainers who provide modifications for all fitness levels.

Using these resources, you can expand your knowledge, stay motivated, and continue exploring ways to maintain an active and healthy lifestyle beyond 50. Remember, the key to long-term success is consistency, enjoyment, and making choices that feel right for you. Happy fitness journey!

ABOUT THE AUTHOR

STAYING PHYSICALLY FIT AT 50 AND BEYOND

Transform Your Body, Transform Your Life: Fitness After 50."

Pastor Anthony Odita is the Senior Pastor and President of Sought-After Believers Ministry. Aka. City Of Royalty in Lagos Nigeria. He is grace with a Unique, Prophetic Anointing to impart and set the captives free. A Teacher, Preacher, Motivational speaker in conferences, a Counsellor, and much sought after among Christian communities. Call by God with a specific mandate to raise royaties. He is blessed to be a blessing to his generation. Married to Pastor Rita Odita and they are blessed with children.

Published by:

Anthony Odita Publications

Open To Invitation.

+234-8143375192

Sought After Believers Ministry International

Sabministry@gmail.com

Email: oditaanthony@yahoo.com